Muscle Building for Men

I0440136

An Introductory Guide to Building Muscle Mass

RON KNESS

Table of Contents

Disclaimer 3

Introduction 4

    The Six Pack – Always a Favorite 7

    Strong Shoulders Will Get You Noticed..............................9

    A Big Chest, But Only When Done Right..........................10

    Upper Back – Make Yourself Look As Good Walking Away...11

    Develop Arms to Hold Her Tight 12

    The Butt – Oh Yeah Baby! 13

    Complete the Package With Strong Legs 13

    Create Your Muscle Building Plan....................................15

What Muscle Type Are You? 16

    The Ectomorph Muscle 17

    Your Problem Areas 19

    Workout Routine, Schedule and Nutritional Needs 19

    The Endomorph Muscle 20

    Your Problem Areas 22

    Workout Routine, Schedule and Nutritional Needs 22

    The Mesomorph Muscle..23

    Your Problem Areas 24

    Workout Routine, Schedule and Nutritional Needs 25

Tailor Your Muscle Build to Your Sport 27

Golf 27

Walking or Running 29

Rowing 31

Volleyball 32

Basketball 34

Football 35

Soccer 37

After Workout Recovery 39

Why Do My Muscles Hurt After A Workout? 40

How to Treat Sore Muscles After A Workout 42

The Plan – How to Create Your Individualized Muscle Building Workout Schedule 44

Diet – An Important Component to Building Muscle 46

In the End 49

About the Author 51

Disclaimer

All the material contained in this book is provided for educational and informational purposes only. No responsibility can be taken for any results or outcomes resulting from the use of this material.

While every attempt has been made to provide information that is both accurate and effective, the author does not assume any responsibility for the accuracy or use/misuse of this information.

Use this information at your own risk.

.

Introduction

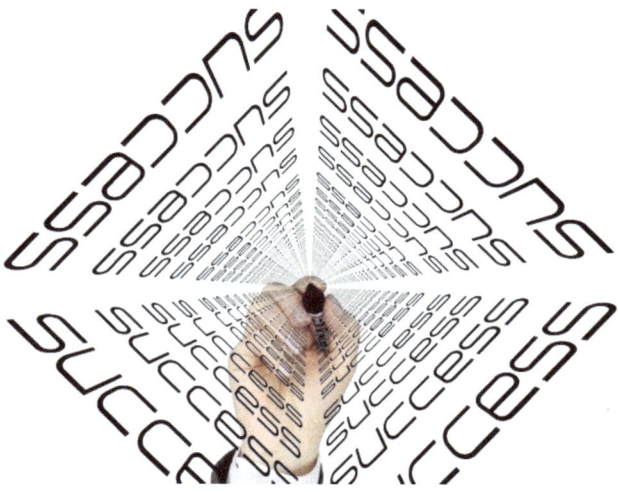

When you start a muscle building program, be aware that this has generally has been a male sport. That doesn't mean that females can't be muscle builders, but male muscle building has always been the norm. The reasons are far reaching actually.

Males naturally produce a large amount of testosterone in their bodies. Testosterone lends itself to longer, more intense workouts. It's a natural part of male muscle building. Testosterone makes men more aggressive, and as a result, they are able to work out more intensely. That means their muscles work harder and grow larger because of their muscle building program.

When the talk begins to turn toward male muscle building, it's natural to speak of muscle building supplements. Many males can benefit from muscle building supplements just as many females can. However, because of the male anatomy as well as the naturally produced hormones by men, they can benefit much more by adding supplements to their workout programs.

Males are better able to focus on muscle building because of their natural constitutions. Their muscles are just waiting to be worked to the point of toned as opposed to females. That's not to say that females are not able to work out with the same intensity as males. What it means is that men grow differently that women do and so do their muscles.

When males are undertaking a muscle building program, they need to keep in mind a few specific points. Among these include maintaining an adequate diet that will give you the vitamins and minerals that you need to bring the nutrition to your muscles that will help you to build muscle mass.

An effective male muscle building program also needs lots of rest as well as lots of water intake. You need to hydrate yourself along with your muscles to make sure that the water works for the good of your workout.

Muscle building for males means working muscles beyond what you ever thought they could do. As a male, you are naturally able to build your muscles because of the hormones that you produce. That makes you at an advantage over the women, but not always. The effectiveness of a workout depends on how hard you work your muscles and how you concentrate your energy.

Muscle building for males requires you to concentrate on certain muscle groups so that you can make some huge muscle mass. If that is your goal as a male muscle builder, then by all means, pursue it! Male muscle building means making a gorgeously toned muscle while becoming fit and trim at the same time.

What Muscles Do Women Like On a Man?

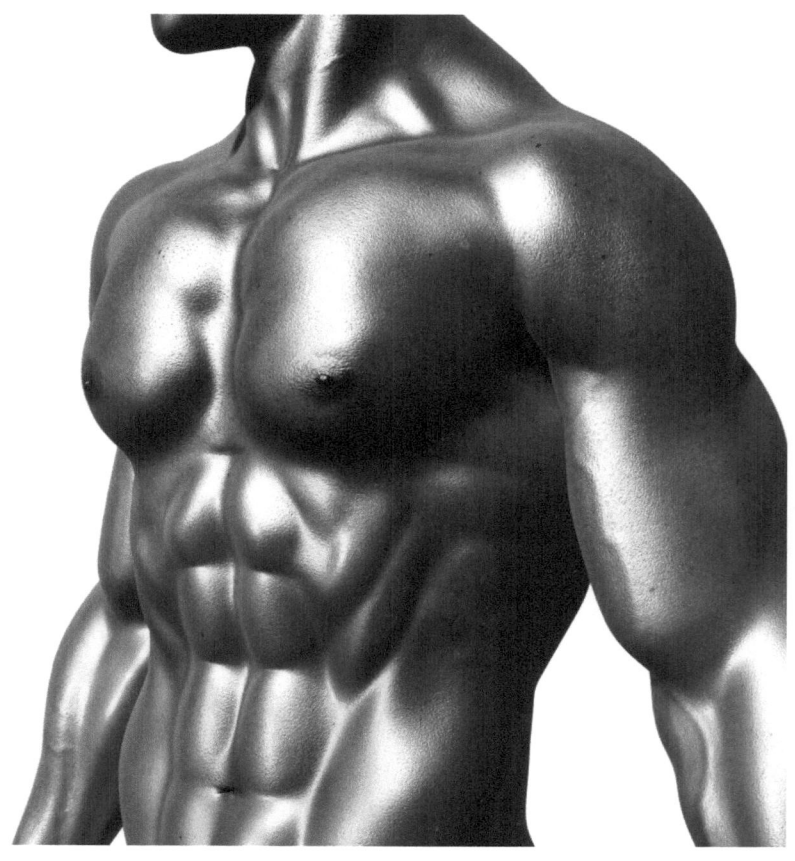

Men and women think very differently about a lot of things –
but both sexes can appreciate a fit muscle. The problem is
that men don't really understand what women want in terms
of muscles on a man – or which muscles even matter.

A chiseled muscle is attractive – and you should work on an all-over toning regimen so that you're not left with one area that's built right and the rest of your body in a flimsy shape.

Every woman will give you a different answer as to what her favorite muscle of the male body is. Some will be attracted to a set of six pack abs, while others have eyes that head straight for the butt.

You want to make sure you have a great well-toned physique so that your muscle is attractive to all of the women you want to meet – and so that you exude confidence when you're out at the pool or elsewhere she might see your muscles.

The Six Pack – Always a Favorite

There's no denying the fact that women love a flat, carved out stomach on a guy. Whether she sees it on the beach or in a more intimate setting, she will love seeing a zero-flab tummy with a set of stacked abs.

This part of a man can be even more amplified for sexiness if he works on the specific V-Cut. This is the lower ab area that literally looks like a V right above the groin.

When a man is wearing swim trunks that are low, you can see the chiseled feature and it shows there's not an ounce of fat on his muscle (not the bad kind, anyway).

Some guys focus so much on chest and back muscles (or legs) that they leave their stomach all flabby. Even if you're not carrying a stomach that makes you look like you have a bun in the oven, if it's just a soft flat stomach, that's not as sexy as carved abs are.

To achieve this look, you have to have a good combination of diet and exercise. You can exercise all you want, but if you eat nothing but junk food, you'll find it hard to keep fat from piling up on your stomach.

When you start working on carving out this area of your stomach, you'll notice that the V-cut is hardest to achieve. You'll get the six pack of abs before the V-cut makes an appearance – and if you start slacking at the gym or on your diet, it'll disappear quickly.

Work on improving your diet to eliminate the fat stores on your muscle, but also go ahead and begin tightening your abs so that as soon as the fat melts off, women will be able to see the six pack forming. It does not good if you have a well-defined six-pack if it is hid under a layer of belly fat.

While we're on the subject, nothing goes better with a six pack of abs than a shaved chest and stomach. A six-pack covered in hair is just a complete turn off for most women.

Strong Shoulders Will Get You Noticed

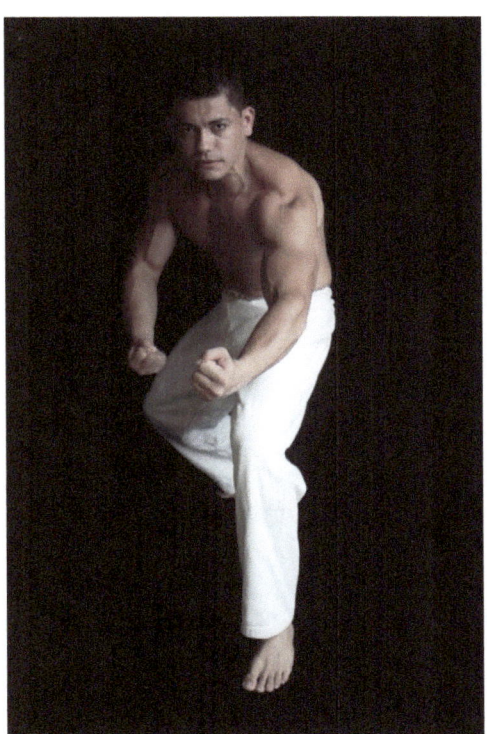

They're not something more women consciously realize they're attracted to, but when you compare pictures of the men women feel are hot to those they feel are weak and unattractive, shoulders are undeniably on the list of must-have muscles.

Now before you go trying to turn into The Hulk, stop and realized that tones and chiseled does not mean bulky and boulder-like. Women want someone who has strength and fitness, but he doesn't have to be able to lift a car.

Shoulder muscles make women instantly think about all of those movie scenes where men come in the room, sweep them off their feet and carry them into the bedroom.

A guy with weak shoulder muscles can't do that. He'd have to point her to the room and follow along behind. It's just not the same. You want to work on strengthening your shoulders without amassing too much size so that it makes it look like you've lost your neck in all those muscles.

Women see strong shoulders as a sign of security. They'll love it when you wrap your big, strong arms around them and hold them – so you want to show that off and let them know you're a source of support and comfort.

When she looks at you and sees strong shoulders, she's instantly picturing herself laying her head on your shoulder at night – and she doesn't want bony or a cushion of fat covering that up.

How do you achieve sexy shoulders? You want them a little wide, which really works great when you have a slim waist (like an upside-down pyramid). You can do specific shoulder exercises using your muscle weight or machines at the gym, but again, you need to pair this with a lean diet.

One other way that working on your shoulders attracts women is because strong shoulders help you have a better posture. A better posture, walking upright instead of slouching, makes her believe you're more confident – and confidence is very attractive to all women.

A Big Chest, But Only When Done Right

Guys often love it when a girl has a nice, big chest. But when it comes to what women want in a man, a big chest better not mean man boobs! Hairy, flabby chests aren't something that makes women drool – so you have to slim down, tone up and carve out the right muscles.

During sexual encounters, if a woman is on top, this is the part of your muscle that she's seeing and touching, so you want to work on this carefully. Use tanning lotion or naturally tan, and shave your chest for stronger appeal.

You don't want to bulk up so much that you're nothing but chest. Women like toned muscles, a little bit of bulk, but not so many muscles that you look like a massive boulder standing in front of them.

Use dumbbells and bodyweight exercises (like dips and pushups) to help chisel out your chest and beef it up a little. Work on building up your pectoral muscles, and that, combined with your shoulder and ab routine, should give you a great upper muscle appeal.

Upper Back – Make Yourself Look As Good Walking Away

You don't want to be carved only on one side. You want to look as good going as you do coming, so you need to address the backside of your upper muscle. Back muscles also help with your posture and confidence generation.

It helps form the upside-down triangle look, and if you're on the skinny side, working on your back muscles can help you look bigger than you actually are in the chest area.

You want to work on all of your back muscles – for different reasons. Your workout strategy on the latissimus dorsi is going to be the muscle that leaks into the sides of the upper muscle – making you appear bigger and stronger.

Don't ignore the deltoids and trapezius – those help you bulk up a bit, but don't go too far so that you lose your entire neck to a large, hulking back. Don't forget your lower back muscles, either. The obliques and rectus abdominus will help you stand taller and straighter, emitting a sense of confidence and appeal to the women you're around.

Develop Arms to Hold Her Tight

Your biceps and forearms are two drool-worthy parts of your muscle that you're going to want to work on. You work with your arms, and women love to see the carved muscle flexing as you lift items, work, etc.

For some women, the biceps and forearms are the top part of a man's muscle. They imagine them hold them in an embrace and being able to handle hard work that needs to be done.

Don't just work on one or the other, though. Strengthen both of them, instead. Make sure they're tanned, too – and always have clean hands, even if the work you do makes them rough. Don't go out with dirty fingernails because it will ruin all of the work you put into building attractive arm muscles.

Show off your arms by not always covering them up with long sleeves. You can layer your clothes if it's cold, and then wear short sleeves to show them off. There's no need to beef up like an over-filled balloon – just pump them up enough so they appear well maintained.

If your arms are tiny, then you may need to work on building muscle mass to get them built up a little. You can't spot train your arms and expect them to grow in size – you have to work your back and add mass for them to fill out nicely.

Make sure you're not overworking your biceps and forearms (through other exercise routines you're doing) because then it eliminates any rest for those muscles, and they won't have a chance to grow.

The Butt – Oh Yeah Baby!

There are many guys who say they're into how a woman's butt looks – and many women who feel the same about the men they're checking out. You don't want to have a bad butt.

One that's saggy or flat can be a big turn off to a woman – even if the rest of your muscle is nice and toned for her. Sometimes, you can get some help with your butt appeal from your clothes – primarily to camouflage it.

But in some clothes, and especially when you're not wearing any clothes, you need to rely on your muscles to make it look appealing. Ladies love for a man to have a nice butt when he's wearing a pair of tight fitting jeans.

Levi jeans are perfect for men who want to attract a woman who appreciates a well-rounded, tight butt. But you have to do your part and get into the gym and work on it, too.

You want to use a combination of squats, lunges, pelvic lifts and other exercises to help firm and increase the size of your buttocks. And if you happen to know you have a hairy bum, make sure you remedy that before an intimate situation arises.

Complete the Package With Strong Legs

Some guys go to the gym and create a great upper muscle – or they focus only on legs and end up having bulky tree trunks that turn a woman off. You want to have a middle of the road approach.

If your legs are fat and flabby, then you need to burn off the fat and firm them up. If they're looking like chicken legs, then you need to amass some bulk on your muscle so that it will flesh them out a bit.

Many women don't care about legs as long as they're normal and average. You don't have to have chiseled, perfectly structured leg muscles. But if they go to one extreme to the other (fat or skinny), then that's where you'll run into trouble.

She wants to look at you and see an overall snapshot of good physical health and fitness. Your calves and hamstrings and quads should all be toned nicely and look like they have a bit of muscle for support and strength.

Your calves and thighs should be tanned and you don't have to shave your legs. In fact, shaving your legs (if you're a runner or swimmer, for instance) can be a turn off to some women who think it makes you look too feminine.

Some women like to see men's calves and dislike seeing men wear short shorts – even if his calves are good. Look for whatever is in style and go with that kind of apparel.

Work on your calves by doing calf raises, but also do lunges, curls and dead lifts and leg presses to help give your lower muscle an all over workout that strengthens and tones your legs.

Create Your Muscle Building Plan

Even if you know a specific woman who likes a certain part of the muscle and you're trying to look attractive to her, spot training usually doesn't work too well. Your best bet is to formulate an all-over workout routine that helps you do three things:

- Burn fat

- Build muscle mass

- Strengthen your muscle

Eliminate hair from your back, buttocks and chest – you can leave the rest, and use a safe option to help you achieve a tan muscle so that your newly carved muscles don't look pasty white.

What Muscle Type Are You?

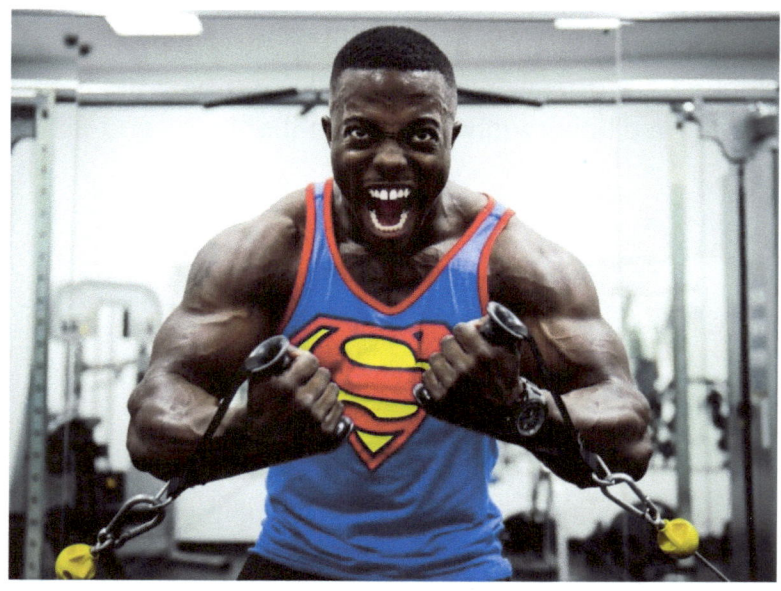

Not all bodies are identical, so choosing a cookie cutter muscle-building plan is a recipe for disaster. You want results, and the best way to get them is to tailor a plan to your specific needs.

You may have tried to build muscle in the past, but without much success. The problem probably wasn't you. It was the plan you were using.

There are three main muscle types you need to know about when you want to build muscle - and you need to know which category you fit into so that you can choose the best and fastest way to put on muscle.

The three main muscle types are Ectomorph, Endomorph and Mesomorph. We'll break down each muscle type so you can understand the strengths and problem areas you might encounter as well as the ways you can thwart any roadblocks to your success.

The Ectomorph Muscle

An ectomorph muscle means that you have the leanest frame of all the muscle types. It can be harder (but not impossible) for someone with this muscle type to build muscle. There are ways that you can tell if this title describes you.

First, your bone structure will be small boned. Sometimes people with this type of muscle will appear to be lean or even underweight. Long arms and legs are associated with this muscle type.

If you're a woman, you won't be rounded - your build will have an almost boyish frame. Women with an ectomorph muscle often have flatter chests and rear ends.

You can look back at your years growing up to pinpoint if you fit this description. Most men and women who fit the ectomorph muscle type will have been very thin as a child. You may have been very active as a child and as an adult, eat a healthy, balanced diet and still struggle to gain weight.

The struggle to gain weight is because your metabolism is faster than those with other muscle types. You may feel you eat a lot of food - in fact, others may have commented that you eat and eat and never gain weight.

Another clue that this is your muscle type is if your appearance doesn't fit your age. You can appear several years to a decade younger than you actually are. You might be someone who's often asked for ID to prove your age.

Those with ectomorph bodies are often narrow shouldered and sometimes even have shoulders that bow inward giving the chest a concave appearance.

Being tall can also be a clue that your muscle is an ectomorph muscle. You can also do a quick check to see if you fit this category. Circle your wrist with your middle finger and thumb. If your finger and thumb overlap, that means your muscle type is ectomorph.

Knowing that you have an ectomorph muscle is just the beginning. You might be happy with your lean frame, but you hate that you look fragile. If you're a man, this might be more of a struggle to deal with than it is for a woman because men often associate being fragile looking with being weaker.

However, if you're a woman and you feel your muscle type makes you look boyish, then you may want to put on muscle in order to give your muscle the curves you want it to have.

You may be completely happy with having an ectomorph muscle type, but you want to gain some weight without it being fat weight. The right muscle building plan can help you gain muscle weight at a healthy pace.

Your Problem Areas

For an ectomorph muscle, one of the problems when trying to build muscle is that the metabolism is so fast that many types of workouts will have the opposite effect.

You'll lose weight because you burn fuel so fast. You end up with a muscle mass index lower than you should have.

Another problem is that people with an ectomorph muscle follow a general workout routine on top of trying to build muscle and on top of other activities such as swimming, jogging, etc.

If you want to build muscle, you have to scale way back on any activity that can make you lose weight like cardio training. Instead, focus on following a structured strength building or weight lifting workout routine.

Workout Routine, Schedule and Nutritional Needs

You would think that cardio is always a great workout for any muscle, but for an ectomorph, a little goes a long way. If this is your muscle type, you can't engage in a lot of high paced cardio workouts like running or aerobics when you're trying to bulk up.

Your focus should be two areas: strength training and eating. Your workouts should consist of routines that build muscles for your shoulders, arms, legs, back and chest. You need to focus on raises, presses and rows as well as curls, squats, barbells and bench presses.

You'll want to work out using machines as well as free weights. Do 2-4 sets with a 1 to 2 minute rest time between sets. The reps will vary according to the area of the muscle you're working out.

Your nutritional needs are extremely important. You need to consume 500 or more extra calories every day. You should eat 5-6 times a day and pack those meals full of lean protein.

If you don't eat enough and then you work out to build muscle, you're going to end up disappointed. If you have an ectomorph muscle type, you have to eat a lot - even if you don't want to.

Some people with this muscle type also take nutritional supplements to help gain weight, but if you concentrate on adding more healthy calories to your everyday meals, you won't have to take a supplement.

The Endomorph Muscle

Many men and women find themselves in the endomorph muscle type category. An endomorph means this is a person who happens to have a higher fat to muscle ratio and the appearance is more rounded.

People with this muscle type can easily become obese if the weight gain isn't stopped. You can tell that you're an endomorph type if you circle your middle finger and thumb around your wrist and the tips can't touch.

If you're a woman with an endomorph muscle, you'll have wider hips and be curvier. Even though curves can be a good thing, on your muscle frame, it will give you a heavier appearance. Women with a pear shaped muscle fit into this category.

If you're a man with an endomorph muscle, you can be described as stocky - which may or may not make you look heavier than you really are. There are certain characteristics that can help you define if this is your muscle type.

First, you'll be a big boned person. You'll be plump or noticeably overweight. Your waist will be higher than the average person's and your metabolism will be slow. You may have dieted in the past and found it difficult to lose weight.

For people with this muscle type, their weakness is the ability to gain weight quickly. However, the thing that works in their favor when building muscle is that they have strong muscles to begin with. People with strong muscles do extremely well with revving up their strength training routines.

One of the reasons that people with an endomorph muscle want to build muscle is to change their muscle appearance from one of softness to one of physical strength. Another reason is that people with this muscle type have a tendency to carry weight around the stomach area and want to change that for aesthetic and health reasons.

Your Problem Areas

Because your metabolism is slower, your workouts are going to have to be different. Your metabolism is going to make turning the fat into firm muscles a bit of a battle, so the first thing you're going to have to have is dedication.

You must commit yourself to a dedicated muscle building routine and you have to commit yourself to sticking with it for as long as it takes.

Most people who have the endomorph muscle shape find the struggle to be in their legs, rear end and stomach. Particularly, some people can have short, wide legs, and shorter trunks - and adding too much muscle can cause the person to look overly bulked up.

Workout Routine, Schedule and Nutritional Needs

Since your metabolism is slower, you have to have your workouts focused on two main points. You need them to have more repetitions and you need them more often. You should set as your goal as 10-12 reps for all your muscle building sets.

Unlike people with the ectomorph muscle, where the focus should be mainly on building muscle and weight training, people with an endomorph muscle should engage in other high intensity workouts - especially cardio.

These should be between 3-4 times a week and should be a minimum of 45 minutes per workout. Aerobic classes are good for endomorph muscle types, as are treadmill workouts.

You have to work out more often and you have to do it faithfully. You need to focus on fat burning exercises in order to help you build muscle. Out of 7 days in the week, for you, 4 of them should be focused on muscle building. You should have a day of rest from all workouts each week.

Your muscle building routine should focus on an area by breaking it down into days and then shaking up the routine. For example, on the first day of week one, work on your chest. The next day, work on biceps, the following day, work on cardio and so on. You have to have an intense workout in order to build muscle and get rid of the softness.

Make sure you incorporate bench presses, barbells, squats, leg presses, curls and raises in your repetitions.

The Mesomorph Muscle

If you have a mesomorph muscle, then count yourself very fortunate. This definition means you have a muscle that's lean and athletic. It means that it won't be difficult for you to build muscle.

By nature, if you're a mesomorph you'll be stronger than most people.

You can use the wrist bone measuring check to see if you fit this category. When you circle your middle finger and thumb around your wrist, if they can touch, that means you're most likely a mesomorph muscle. Your bones will be medium.

It's also easy to tell if you fit this category because you'll have muscles that are easy to define from fat. However, if you do put on weight, you'll end up looking like you're a lot heavier than you actually are because you have more muscle mass. More muscle mass combined with weight gain makes you look bigger.

When you do decide to work on building muscle, it will happen easily and others may remark on your 'overnight' firmer muscle.

If you're a woman who fits the label of mesomorph, then you'll usually have an hourglass shape and your muscle fat will be spread throughout your muscle rather than gathering in one area.

If you're a man who fits the label, then you'll have broad shoulders and even if you do gain weight, you won't look fat - you'll just look big boned. Both men and women in this category usually have very good posture.

Your Problem Areas

The biggest problem that people with mesomorph bodies have is that they can gain weight so fast. In fact, of the three, this is the easiest muscle type for gaining weight. But it's true that people in this category also have an easier time losing that gain.

Because of their bone structure and strength, people in this category often easily overwork their muscle when building muscle. They have a high capacity for building muscle and a high perseverance level. This drive can easily lead to over training.

Workout Routine, Schedule and Nutritional Needs

Besides being blessed the ideal muscle type, mesomorph people do really well with any kind of resistance training. They have a metabolism that's right in the middle of the three muscle types. Not too fast, and not too slow.

On the downside, though, your muscle can quickly adjust to your muscle building workout - so that means you have to keep it changed up in order to build the muscle and maintain.

Even though you can easily go longer than other people can when working out, you should never push your muscle building workouts longer than an hour. Stick to 45 minutes maximum.

Your workout should consist of moderate weights, since it's easier for you to build muscle. You can set up a workout plan so that you work out every day with one rest day - but every other day will work well for your muscle type. Each set that you do (don't do any more than 5 sets) should have no more than 12 repetitions.

Because an unbalanced diet can lead to fast weight gain for you, try to stick to carbs that are low on the glycemic index and eat plenty of protein. You want to use the 40/30/30 rule. Your carbs should make up 40% of your diet, protein 30% and fat 30%.

If you weighed 200 pounds and needed to consume 400 more calories for your muscle building, then you would eat 340 carbs, 255 grams of protein and 113 grams of fat.

Since that's too much to consume just by eating breakfast, lunch and dinner, you're going to want to break that down by eating more often. Have 5-6 meals throughout the day. It keeps your insulin level under control and helps your metabolism.

Building muscle doesn't have to be a struggle. Once you know what your muscle needs, it will be much easier to accomplish than previous times when you may have been attempting to use a cookie cutter approach.

Tailor Your Muscle Build to Your Sport

Generalized muscle building will help anyone develop muscle mass. But targeted muscle building can help you build muscle that's specifically suited to the sport that you enjoy doing.

When you work to build muscles in the area that's used most often for your sport this will help you to not only gain stamina and speed, but elevate your performance record as well.

Golf

While golf seems like a quiet, relaxed game that's not too

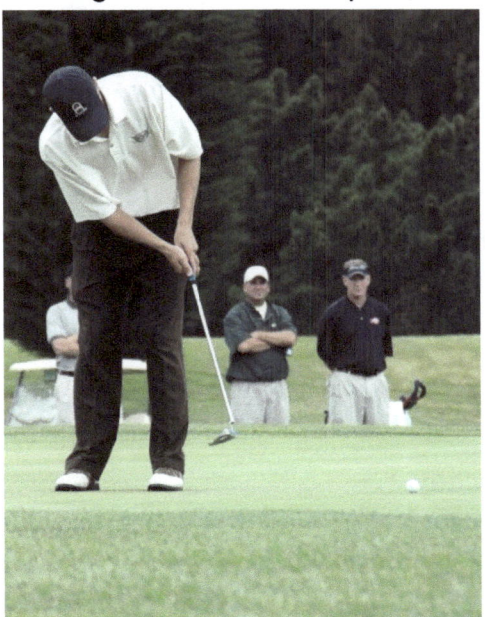

demanding on the muscles of your muscle, you might be surprised to learn that it's anything but that. In fact, golf is a game that uses many different muscle groups.

Playing golf uses muscles from your upper to your lower body. It calls for players to use their chest or prectoralis muscles. But you also use your forearms as well as your back and core muscles.

Your gluteus maximus or butt muscles are instrumental in helping your golf performance, too. It might not seem like it, but it's these muscles that will help the most in improving your golf swing and help you gain distance with your shots.

That's because these muscles are responsible for your posture and the way that you move your hips during play. Your chest and back muscles are the ones used that influence the way that you swing the clubs and whether or not your swing plane stays intact so the ball goes in the direction you want it to.

When you play golf, as you swing your muscle does a rotating movement. This rotating movement is what gives the players power. You'll want strong core muscles, because these muscles are not only your stabilizer, but they also work as your conduits.

They're what transfers the motion from the bottom of your muscle into your torso and back. A lot of people think that playing golf is successful or unsuccessful based on how built someone's arm muscles are.

While it's true that you do need some muscle mass in the forearms to help you with your game, your forearms can only pass on the power from your muscle to put it into the swing.

So if you have weak muscles in the core area or in your gluteus maximus, then that weakness will show up in your swing. Your forearms can't compensate for weak muscles somewhere else in the muscle, and in fact, relying too much on your arms would ruin your game anyway.

You'll want to build muscle in your chest using bench presses with barbells or dumbbells as well as using pushups. To build muscle in the forearms, use a farmer's carry using dumbbells.

You can also do the farmer's carry with kettlebells. Engage in towel pull-up repetitions and also wrist curls. Building muscle in your back means you'll need to use a routine that calls for you to use barbell deadlifts, chin ups, cable rows, V-bar pulldown and a weight shrug using dumbbells.

These exercises build the trapezius as well as the latissimus dorsi. When you need to build your core muscles, you'll want to perform exercises such as push-ups, hip lifts, plank exercises, squats and lunges.

Building the butt muscles means you'll need to do lunges, squats and step-ups. Doing these exercises will help your golf game because you'll be able to rotate your hips with more power and have that power transfer from the core muscles into the forearms. You'll also gain a better sense of balance.

Walking or Running

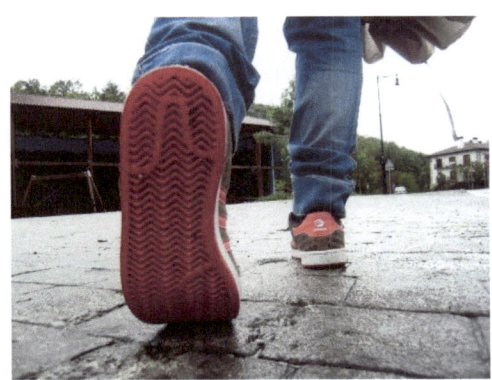

Surprisingly, whether you walk or run, you end up using the majority of your muscle's muscles. When you engage in walking or running as a sport, it's important that you know how to build strength to help you.

The muscles that are used in either sport are identical. You use your abdomen, the calf muscles, your hamstrings, the butt muscles, quadriceps, thighs and hips. You also use your shoulders, biceps and forearms.

Those muscles are the ones that you'll want to concentrate on building up. For the hamstrings, concentrate on deadlifts including one-legged deadlifts using weights.

You'll also want to perform plenty of reps using leg curls. When it comes to building forearm muscles, weights are your friend. Use kettlebells as well as hand weights in varying weight sizes, gradually increasing the weight limit.

Lunges and step-ups are the best way to build up the butt muscles. For the abdomen, it's the use of repetition exercises that will build those muscles. You'll want to do planks, bicycle crunches, ab wheel exercises and sit-ups using weights.

Calf muscles are built using calf raises, both standing and seated, box jumps and jumping squats. Your thigh muscles benefit from squats, lunges and curls. The quadriceps can gain muscle with the use of barbell lunges, barbell squats, bench jumps, and with box and front squats.

The biceps can be built using pushups, arm and squat curls. When you exercise to build the muscles that you use in walking or running, you gain a lot more besides just endurance that can help you last for whatever event you're training to take part in.

You can increase the speed in which it takes you to cover a distance. Because controlling your breathing is invaluable during walking or running to keep you from getting winded, using the exercises specific for these sports can increase your respiratory function.

Rowing

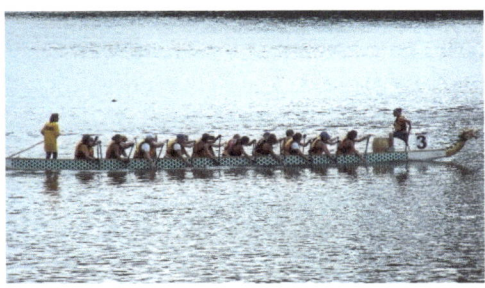 Rowing for sport requires precision and strength. The sport is separated into classes for competition and is an Olympic sport. You have to do more than simply be in good physical shape to row for sport.

You need to have or know how to build muscle in the major muscle groups that you'll be using. In this sport, you'll use your biceps and quadriceps as well as your back and shoulders.

You'll also use your hamstrings and butt muscles as well as your core muscles. It's important that you have and maintain all over muscle fitness, but for rowing, you'll really need to focus on the muscles that will impact your performance.

To build strong muscles in those areas, there are certain exercises you'll want to make a regular part of your routine. You'll want to use deadlifts and squats because these build your hamstrings as well as your butt muscles.

Have plenty of bench press repetitions on the schedule for helping to build the back and shoulder muscles. You need a lot of upper muscle strength in rowing and bench presses can help you obtain that.

Your biceps handle a lot during rowing. Build up those muscles with plenty of curls. All of the muscles that you'll work out play an important role in rowing. You need to build them up for strength and stamina.

Working out the biceps gives you strength in your grip. Exercises that work out your hamstrings help give you stability during rowing. Building muscle in your core muscles help you increase your timing when you push back as you row. It can increase your drive through the water against the resistance.

Volleyball

Playing volleyball is a fun sport, but it's a lot more demanding on the muscle that it first appears to be. Members who play this sport end up working out almost every major muscle group in their muscle.

It's also a sport that's incredibly demanding. This means that it can be hard on the muscles and the joints if you're not working on building up the muscles that are used during play.

The muscles that are used during volleyball include the shoulder and chest as well as the abdomen and back. The hip flexors and butt muscles are used, too - along with the quads, hamstrings and calves.

To play volleyball as a sport, you have to have great core strength. So your workout should consist of exercises that

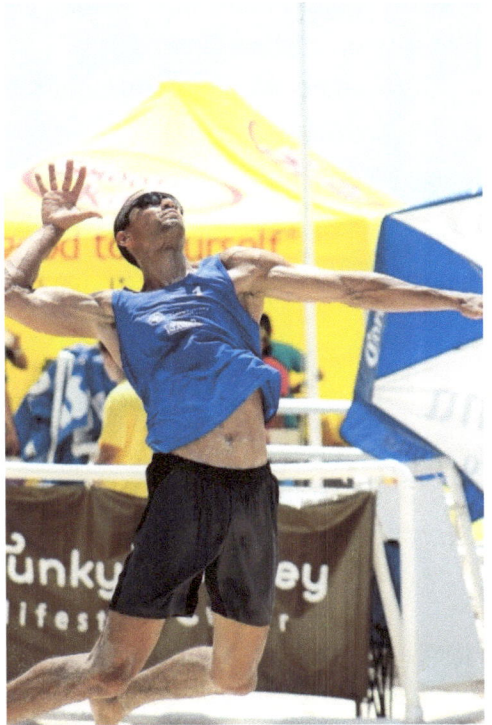

target all of your major muscle groups. Your quads, hamstrings and calves need raises, squats and lunges to build muscle.

Your butt muscles are your muscle's biggest muscle and they need step-up exercises as well as butt lifts and kneeling squats. For the shoulder and chest area muscles, you'll want to do shoulder presses, laterals and push-ups.

The abdomen needs side crunches, prone plank exercises and squats while the back needs a workout routine that includes deadlifts, pull-ups and chin-ups and leg curls.

In volleyball, you have to make a move in a split second and you never know what that move is going to be. By working out the muscles needed in volleyball, you can increase your performance.

Building muscle in the legs gives you the necessary power and thrust that you need when moving to block. Building the muscles also helps to keep you off the injured list.

Basketball

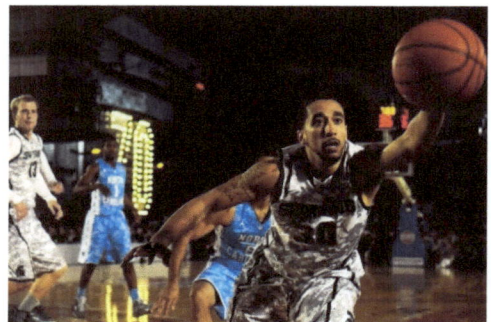

Basketball is another sport that uses the majority of the muscle's muscles. But there are some that it primarily relies on. These muscles are the quads, calves and hamstrings - along with the shoulder, upper chest and arm muscle, such as the triceps and biceps.

The abdominal muscles are used along with the lower back muscles. Players use their legs a lot during play for making the moves that they need to get the ball, shoot the ball and run down the court.

The thigh muscles give players lift while the calves work to tightly control the movement, whether out and out running or short sprints. To get the ball where it needs to be, the triceps are instrumental.

Your effort to get the ball into the basket will be weak if the triceps aren't fully conditioned. When it comes to going on the offensive, you'll need your shoulders and chest area to take the blocks and get to the basket.

You have to make sure that you have plenty of muscle built in your core because these muscles help you quickly dart around other players and make sharp moves when you need to dart one direction or another.

Exercises to build muscle for playing basketball are made up of ones that work the entire muscle. The purpose of these exercises is to build strength and stamina. You'll need to do chin-ups and high pulls as well as front squats.

Lunges need to be a part of your workout, as do push-ups and bench presses. You'll want to do step-ups, but while you're doing these, make sure that you're using dumbbells to increase the strength and shooting capacity of your biceps.

When you play basketball, you must be able to defensively block, take a shoulder hit from another player, shoot from long or short distances and move down court in a second. By building the major muscles, your playing skill will increase.

Football

Football is one of those sports that puts the muscle through a tough series of motions. The sport is strenuous enough so that your entire muscle gets a workout during play.

That means that you have to work on building muscle in both the upper as well as the lower muscle. You need to strengthen and add mass to your hamstrings as well as your butt muscles, because these are used to push forward during the various plays.

You'll be doing a lot of running - and that calls for some serious leg movements. The quadriceps need to be strengthened, because you use these to move your knees.

The chest muscles need to be built to give you the strength 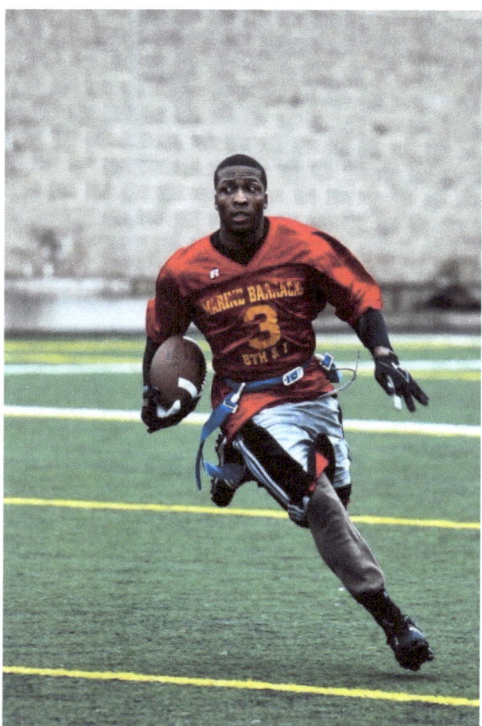 you need to stand strong against an opposing player. Your shoulder muscles are used during plays to get the ball down the field or to another player and the abdominal muscles are used to help maintain your stability.

The triceps give you range of motion for throwing and blocking plays. You have to have strong core muscles, because these allow you the freedom of movement as you leap and turn to catch a pass.

To build your muscles into football ready shape, you need to concentrate on compound exercises, because these give you muscle growth in both the upper and the lower muscle.

When you use compound exercises, you gain build at the same time over using isolation exercises. You need to include squats as well as bench presses in your routine. Also have snatches as part of your compound exercises, because these help with faster muscle contractions.

Soccer

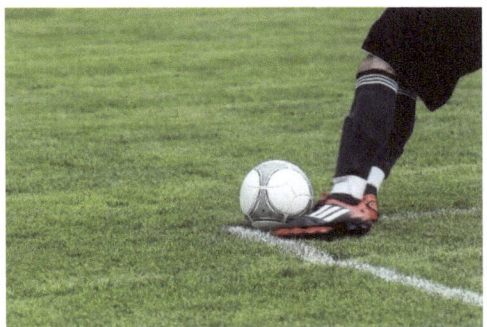 With soccer, you use some of the same muscles that you use in playing football - especially the legs. You'll be using the upper and lower muscle as well. You'll be using the shoulders and the biceps and triceps.

The legs and thighs are the primary muscles used, but so are the core muscles. You need to build muscles in the arms, especially in the shoulders, because these muscles help players maintain balance when they're aiming to head shot the ball.

When it comes to playing soccer, you have to be fast. You also have to be able to maintain control of the ball. Most people assume that the lower leg muscles are the most important part of the leg when it comes to playing soccer, but it's actually the thigh muscles.

These muscles are what provide the player with the speed, control and power needed to kick the ball to a team mate or the goal net. The calf muscle needs to be strong so that players have better foot control when moving the ball. A weak calf muscle will equal poor control over the foot movements.

You want to be cautious when building muscle for soccer, because if you bulk up with too much muscle mass, that can actually slow down your ability to play. You want to concentrate on exercises that make you faster. These will be exercises like split squats, lunges, box jumps and deadlifts.

Building muscle is a wonderful thing to do for anyone who wants to engage in physical fitness. But when it comes to playing sports, not only does it help you achieve your goals in terms of playing the game and scoring, but it helps prevent injuries as well.

After Workout Recovery

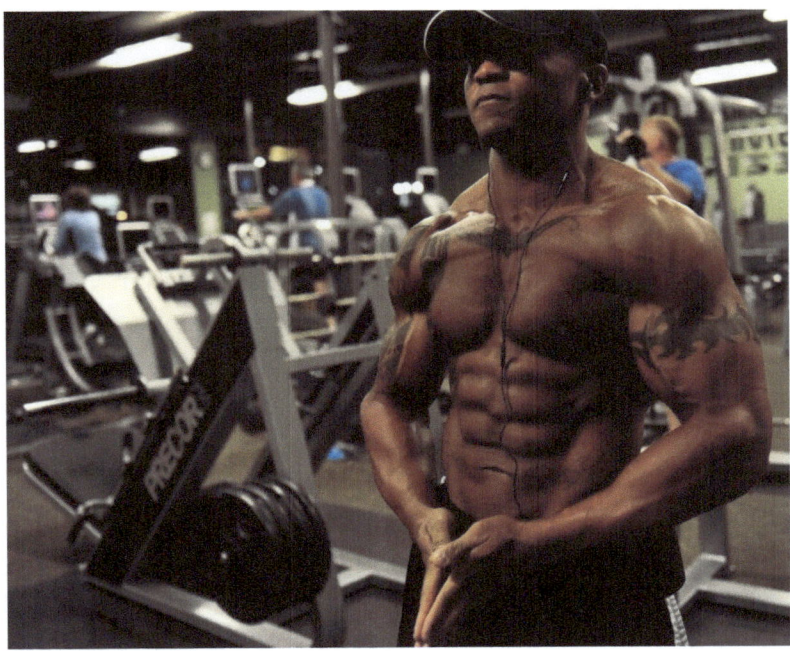

Building muscles is almost an art form of sorts, like sculpting your muscle as an artist would do. Working out your muscle and getting the abs that you want, the stamina that you crave - there's beauty in that - in pushing your muscle to the max to develop the kind of muscle build that's on your goal list.

Building muscle takes dedication and a lot of determination, because after a workout, your muscle can feel like you ran a hundred miles uphill through ankle-deep sludge.

You'll feel the burn in your muscles and sometimes, it can reach the point to where you might start wondering why you even keep going. There's relief at hand for you for those times when your muscles experience the pain of a workout.

Why Do My Muscles Hurt After A Workout?

Anyone wanting to build muscle knows that in order to get the size and cut you're looking for, you must have repetition. This repetition is what strengthens the muscle and causes it to grow.

But, there is a downside to the repetitive moments. When you build muscle, it's putting pressure on the muscles, regardless of what kind of workout you're doing. Using this repeated pressure is what you have to do if you want to see changes in strength as well as a visible difference.

This force is what created the pain that you feel. Though the pain doesn't last for a long time, it's still uncomfortable. When the pain hits you after a muscle building workout, it's called delayed onset muscle soreness - otherwise known as DOMS.

You might have heard the term "no pain, no gain" and when it comes to building your muscles, and it's true. If you're looking to build your muscles or add to your strength ability, you're going to experience some pain.

It's doing the muscle building exercises over and over again that will trigger the pain. The pain is triggered because your muscles get to the point where they reach their max capacity to handle the exercise.

What some people do is once they reach their max capacity, they pull back. If you've reached the muscle size and strength that you want, pulling back will keep you at the size that you currently are right now.

However, if you want to actually *build* the muscle, you have to push past your max capacity and that's when the pain comes. After the workout is over, your muscles will reach a level of fatigue that they didn't have before you started the workout.

During the muscle building process, you went through the repetitions designed to build muscle, and in that time, you had to take the muscles beyond their current comfort zone.

This pain is associated with the stress placed on the muscles during the building phase, but it's especially noticeable if you're new to muscle building. You'll also experience this pain if you're starting a workout that you've never done before or if you're adding new repetitions to a building routine that you currently have.

What happens when the pain hits is that some people assume one of two things. They assume that they did the workout wrong or they assume that they overdid the muscle building, and so they back off or stop for a few days.

The majority of pain isn't associated with an incorrect workout or with overload. The muscles are changing due to the muscle building regimen and any time there's change in the muscle formation, you're going to feel it.

While it can be painful and make you wonder what's going on if you're new to it, pain after a muscle building session doesn't mean that something's wrong. In fact, it might mean you're doing everything right.

How to Treat Sore Muscles After A Workout

If you experience sore muscles because you worked out, hoping to build your mass, the very worst thing that you can do is to stop working out. By not using the muscles, you can actually cause the pain to linger.

It's okay, however, to dial back the intensity of your muscle building workout for a day or so, but you don't want to stop altogether, even for a brief period. When you keep on working out, pushing through the pain, your muscles will warm up and provide you with relief from the soreness that you're experiencing.

You can use ice to treat any sore muscles you might experience from your muscle building workouts. Traditional treatment calls for placing ice on the area that's causing you pain. However, you can also take an ice bath.

This treatment is favored by athletes and involves sitting in an ice bath for no longer than five minutes. The coolness of the temperature reduces the inflammation in the muscles and gives you relief from the pain.

On the flip side of using cold methods to treat sore muscles, you can use heat. With this method of treating sore muscles, you can apply a heating pad directly to the area that's causing you to feel pain.

One of the items that you can use to apply heat is a heating pad or a rice heating bag that you can heat up in the microwave. You can also use heat wraps. You can find these that are made to fit specific areas of the muscle such as the arms, wrists, shoulders, back, neck, knees and ankles.

Anti-inflammatory medication can also be used to help treat the sore muscles you might encounter after a workout. The medicine works by lessening the inflammation that you might have in the muscle that can contribute to the pain.

You can take these types of medication by mouth or you can use them topically through the use of anti-inflammatory patches that can be applied directly on the skin right over the sore muscle.

Sometimes, a massage can also help to reduce or eliminate the pain you'll feel from sore muscles after a muscle building routine. A massage is known to reduce inflammation in muscles. Plus, getting one can give muscle recovery a boost.

While treatment is an option for you, it's best to avoid soreness as much as possible simply because it's not fun. You can avoid most soreness if you make sure that you don't stick too long with one muscle building routine.

When you stick with one routine for too long, your muscles aren't acclimating to any change. So when you do change, you end up sore because you're putting new stress on your muscle.

It's best to change up your routine with a variation of muscle building exercises, rather than getting too comfortable with one. Most muscle soreness isn't anything you need to be concerned about.

However, if the soreness is so much that it prevents you from doing your day to day activities at home or at your job, then it's possible it could be an injury rather than simple soreness.

The Plan – How to Create Your Individualized Muscle Building Workout Schedule

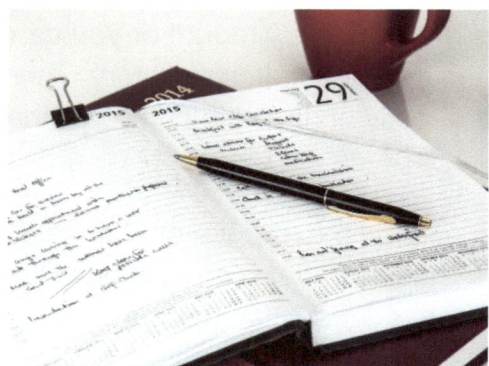

Knowing what muscle group to work out is a must. For the best muscle growth, you'll want to work out each group on a regular and even basis to promote strength.

You'll also have to know when it's time to add more repetitions and more weight to any of your routines. If you're just now starting to build muscle, you'll want to do it gradually and slowly increase your time and repetition.

Otherwise, too much, too soon can lead to muscle injury or burnout. On your muscle building schedule, the first thing that you're going to want to do is to boost the equipment weight that you're using.

You'll want to do this on a regular schedule. Your routine should always progress until you reach the muscle mass that you want to have and maintain. Remember that if you can do the muscle building routine that you've been using comfortably, then it's time to boost your muscles into overdrive, because this is what will build them up.

Adding more weight is one thing to have in the schedule. The amount of repetitions that you'll want to do is another. Once you can blow through the repetitions in your routine, it's time to add to them.

Raise the number of times you perform each set. You should be able to feel the effort - and if it's effortless, then keep adding reps. Another think that you want to do with your muscle building schedule is to make sure that each of the muscle groups are getting a max workout.

That means that you should be working out at least three times a week. As often as you can with your workout schedule, do compound exercises. These offer you multiple benefits because you're not just focusing on one or two muscle areas like you do with isolation exercises.

The more muscles that you can work out at once, the faster you'll build the mass that you want to have. You gain strength faster this way, too. You must have recovery built into your schedule, because this is an important factor in building muscles.

The way that you set up your recovery schedule can follow a standard guideline used to build muscle, but it's better if you conform your recovery period based on your own muscle.

Not everyone recovers at the same pace. So your schedule would need to be based on how long it takes your muscle to recover. The recovery phase that you set up should also take into consideration the level of your workout.

This phase is going to be different for someone who engages in moderate muscle building workouts versus someone who works harder. The recovery period for you will also depend on how many days a week you exercise as well as the length of time you give each of your workout sessions.

You should also factor in your diet. The amount of meals that you consume, plus the calories can matter in a recovery schedule. Plus the types of food you have and the times that you eat these foods also play an important part.

Building muscle takes dedication, but it can also put a lot of stress on you both physically and mentally. Your recovery should be worked into your muscle building schedule based on the load that you think you can withstand.

It's true that muscle building isn't always pleasant, but it shouldn't make you stressed out or make you feel miserable.

Diet – An Important Component to Building Muscle

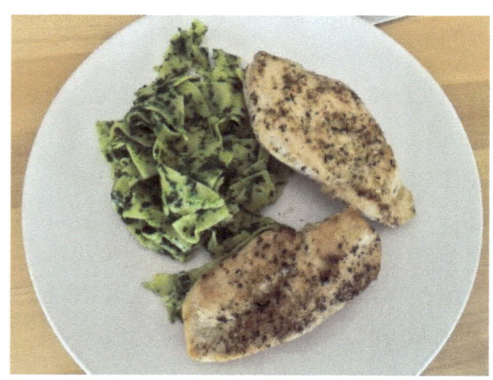

Muscle building takes a lot of calories - more so than any regular muscle exercise, because of the difference in the two. With regular exercise, the focus isn't on creating mass, but rather getting fit and getting or keep the weight off.

With muscle building, you're putting the weight on deliberately as muscle mass, so you have to have the right kind and the right amount of calories as well as nutrients.

Not having the right kind of diet can really work against your goals. Normal advice with calories says not to take in more than you use, but it's the opposite with muscle building.

You have to take in more calories than you use because it's this fuel that your muscle uses to turn it into muscle. If you've ever worked hard to build muscle and haven't been able to, check the amount of calorie intake and raise it significantly and that will help.

If you've already achieved some muscle mass, but you're looking to grow bigger, then add about 500 calories a day to your eating schedule. If you check your progress and discover that you're gaining muscle, then you're doing it right.

If you're packing on flab, then you're doing it wrong. Your diet needs to consist of a whole lot of protein. These are foods like dairy and meat, like chicken and beef. This is essential for building muscle.

The amount of protein that you eat should be figured as grams to muscle weight. For every pound that you weigh, you should eat one gram of protein. You also need to make sure that you cover fats and a lot of carbs in your diet.

Nuts are especially helpful in your diet for helping the muscle build muscle. The amount of carbs that you eat should be figured according to your muscle weight as well.

For each pound of weight that you carry, make sure that you're consuming between 2-3 grams of carbohydrates. Fats are figured a little different than per pound of muscle weight.

For this, you want to be sure that you're dividing by a pound and half of muscle weight for each gram of fat. The amount of calories that you need to consume to build muscle can be broken down any way that you like.

If you prefer to eat more often, just divide your calories that way. Or, if you like the idea of just sticking to breakfast, lunch and dinner, then you can split the calories you have to have between three meals.

Your diet matters during the recovery phase. This is the time right after the workout, and while the last thing you might want to do is eat, you need to let the food help your muscle begin the repair process.

The time frame for you to eat is within the first two hours after you've gone through your muscle building routine. If you're looking to build muscle, then you should see an increase in your weight every week of at least a pound.

When you step on the scale, if you're not seeing this kind of gain, then you need to add to your calorie intake little by little until you're seeing that pound a week gain that you're striving for.

In the End ...

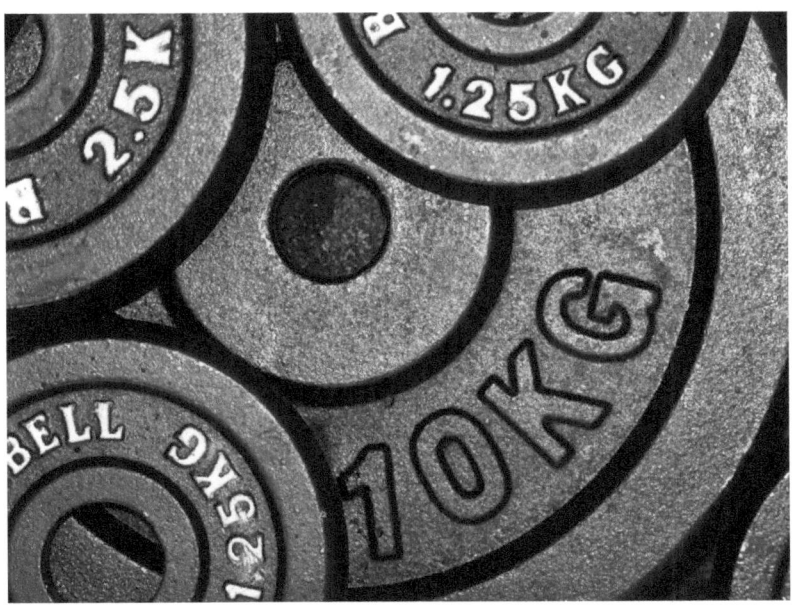

Muscle building isn't for everyone, but we're willing to bet that once you start on a workout program, you'll realize that it's the best thing you've ever done for yourself. You'll look better, you'll feel better, and your confidence will soar. And you'll attract the attention of the opposite sex (if that is the attention you want to notice you).

Many people start out building muscle in an attempt to lose weight. And that's a great way to start. But then, they start learning about what their body is doing during a workout and what it is capable of when pushed. After that door is opened, there's so much to learn and gain (literally).

I remember in my younger years when I would read comic books, in the back of the book, there was always an advertising section. One ad that always caught my eye was the one where the 90 pound weakling went on to become a muscle-bound 160 pound specimen for all to envy.

These results aren't unheard of and can actually be achieved by anyone who is willing to put in the time and effort to do so. You don't have to be satisfied with a body that is less than what you want it to be.

It does take hard work in the gym, eating right and a lot of dedication, but once you start, you'll find yourself wanting to continue more than wanting to stop. When you are finally able to look at yourself in the mirror and like what you see, the end result will be well worth any sacrifice you have made along the way.

Get started right away. You don't have to wait any longer. Your dream body is more than a possibility – it's a reality. So go out and get ripped. There's no time like right now!

About the Author

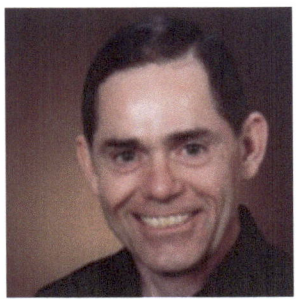

I grew up in Central Minnesota, where my parents own and operated a fishing resort. Once out of high school I tried a couple of semesters of college, only to quit halfway through the Spring term; I decided at that time that college wasn't for me.

Then I decided to follow my father's previous occupation as an auto mechanic. I graduated from a two-year of vocational training course and worked as a mechanic. While in vocational training, I decided to join the National Guard where I eventually ended up working full-time for 32 years.

So how does all of this relate to writing? In one of my leadership schools, the instructor, who was an English teacher at a juvenile detention center, presented writing to me in a whole new way - a way that started to develop my interest in working with words.

Fast forward about 40 years and I now have over 20 books listed on Amazon for Kindle. All of my books with the exception of one children's book (One, Two, Three, Four . . . Counting is Fun at the Grocery Store) are non-fiction in various fields, such as:

*Health and Fitness:

- What You Eat Can Hurt You

- Eat Healthy to Lose Weight

- The Extreme Weight Loss Plan

- Get Ripped Abs

- Walking Down the Road to Fitness

- Design Your Ultimate Fitness Program - Walking

- A Healthier You in the Coming Year

- Senior Fitness – A Guide to Staying Young Beyond Your Years

- Managing Type 2 Diabetes Using Alternative And Natural Therapies

- How Diet and Exercise Can Better Manage Type 2 Diabetes

* Self-Publishing:
- Writing for the Kindle

- How to Self-Publish Your Ebook on Amazon

- Pillars of Gold

- Kindle Advanced Strategies

- Self-publishing - Work Smarter, Not Harder

- The Home-Based Entrepreneur's Guide to Blogging

* Digital Photography:
- The Digital Photography Interactive Quiz

- How to Improve your Travel Photography

- Digital Photography: Aperture, Shutter Speed and You

- Don't Be In the Dark About Light

- The No Nonsense Guide to Digital Photography

- The Beginner's Guide to Digital Photography

- Digital Photography – A Quick Guide to Using Adobe Photoshop Elements

- Improve Your Blog Posts With Photos

- Digital Photography Anthology

* Travel:
- Travel Advisor

- Travel Trips and Tips

*Outdoors and Recreation:

- Making Your First Fly Rod

- The Beginner's Guide to Fly Tying

- Hooked on Fly Fishing

- The Secrets to Fly Fishing for Trout

- Tent Camping – The Ultimate in Family Fun

- Maintaining a Salt Water Pool

* Misc.:
- Making Wine from Kits

- Create Your Home Inventory

- The 9 Secrets to Using Your GI Bill Benefits

- The Life and Times of the Honey Bee

- The Military Spouses Financial Guide to Funding Education

- The Home-Based Entrepreneur's Guide to Blogging

Survival Basics – Are You Prepared to Survive?

Besides my own writing, I also ghostwrite ebooks, reports, articles, blogs and do Kindle conversions for my clients.

Oh . . . did I mention that I went back to college in 1987 and graduated 7 years later?

Today my wife and I live in Gold Canyon, AZ, where you'll find me happily sitting in my office typing away on my laptop as I work on my next book or ghostwriting project . . . that is if we are not traveling on a cruise ship - our new-found mode of travel.

If you like my book, please leave a review of it on Amazon at the book link above.

www.ingramcontent.com/pod-product-compliance
Lightning Source LLC
Chambersburg PA
CBHW050824290526
45792CB00001B/251